MW01269028

COMMON WAYS FOR COMMON PEOPLE

TEAS, BREWS, NOURISHING INFUSIONS.

APRIL GRAHAM

Wildwood

Copyright © 2023 by April Graham

All rights reserved.

No portion of this book may be reproduced in any form without written permission from the publisher or author except as permitted by U.S. copyright law.

CONTENTS

1

INTRODUCTION

I swear, half of the time, I have the stamina to do anything; it's from the gallons of nourishing herbal infusion I drink on a weekly basis.

While I'm sure the food I eat and the sleep I get are part of the reason I have energy, I can for sure say if I don't drink my infusions, I feel a noticeable difference!

Yet, I don't want not to give credit where credit is due when it comes to how much tea also supports me. Although I know with tea, I'm not really after nutrients so much as I am after the more volatile properties.

That may sound odd, so let's break down the differences between nourishing herbal infusions and teas and go from there.

2

WHAT IS A NOURISHING HERBAL INFUSION?

These are when we take a specific weighed-out amount of dried herb, place the herb into a jar, pour boiling water over top, cap, and allow to set between 4-24 hours before we strain out the plant matter.

This long timeframe and the water going from very hot to room temperature allow really high levels of nutrients and medicinal properties out of whatever herb we are working with.

Of course, folks mainly make these to drink, but we can also use them as ingredients in making herbal creations that contain water, like lotions or creams.

We can also use them on our hair, in our bath, soaking our feet, and even to fertilize other plants.

They are absolutely packed with vitamins, minerals, and medicinal properties due to the large amounts of herbs used and the long set time.

3

WHAT IS A TEA?

While I feel pretty sure we all know what tea is, you never really know these days.

Tea is like a nourishing herbal infusion in the way that you need dried herbs and hot water to make it, but tea is usually made with a blend of different herbs, and there is a very small amount of herb(s) per one little teacup or mug.

We often also add sweeteners, and some of us add cream.

These are often allowed to steep in hot water for 5-15 minutes, max.

The main reason for teas is because they are tasty and relaxing, and they help us feel warm. More potent herbs give us some healing actions. We can cook with them and even rinse our hair in them.

These have very few vitamins or minerals and will only have any real worthwhile medicinal value if the herb used is fragrant or has many tannins.

4

When to Choose a Nourishing Herbal Infusion.

If the plant we are working with does not have much of a scent and heals us primarily from her nutritional content, this is an ideal choice for a nourishing herbal infusion.

Take Plantain leaf (not the banana, ha.) as an example.

She has no real smell and is packed with a lot of really amazing vitamins and minerals.

Her medicinal qualities make her ideal for a nourishing herbal infusion.

Whether we are going to be drinking it or using it in some other way, the bigger volume of herb and the longer wait time will ensure we get all we want from her.

WHEN TO CHOOSE A TEA

Teas are best for plants that have a really strong scent, as these plants often don't heal us in the way of nutritional content but really high levels of different volatile oils and other compounds.

This also means that a little goes a very long way.

We don't need a ton of herbs in our hot water, and a long brew time is actually somewhat dangerous.

Lavender is a perfect example here.

She is extremely fragrant, and - while very healing in small amounts - if you made a nourishing herbal infusion out of her and drank it, you could really hurt yourself.

6

WHEN TO KINDA SORTA MAKE BOTH

Because there is never anything in the world that is as cut and dry as we often assume, there are other plants that kinda need to be made like an infusion, but also a tea.

I mean, things like roots and mushrooms should not really be made into a full-on, set-for-24-hour infusion, but it's also pointless to just soak a tiny amount in some hot water for a handful of minutes.

Dandelion root is a good example of this.

If you make a nourishing herbal infusion, you'll probably vomit from drinking it, but if you just let it sit in some hot water for a moment, the water won't even make it all the way to the center of the root pieces.

These herbs - anything that is really pretty firm - need to be actively simmered.

Roots usually need to be simmered for 20-30 minutes, depending on how bitter they are, and most mushrooms need to be simmered for no less than an hour to release their highly prized PSK (Polysaccharide-K) content (which fights cancer).

This is yet another great example of why we need to get to know each plant we are working with - so we can ask ourselves if she is better made in this way or another way?

7

YOU MADE BROTH

I am sorry to say that if you are using fresh plant matter to try and make a nourishing herbal infusion, tea, or simmered-down brew, you made none of these things.

You made a weak broth.

All these things can only be made with dried herbs, and there is a good reason for this!

I want you to picture a really big uncooked potato in your mind.

It's pretty firm, right?

Like, it's so firm that if you threw an uncooked potato at someone as hard as you could, it would not be unreasonable to assume that you could knock someone out, right?

Haha, you just imagined doing that!

Well, some of you did.

Now imagine what would happen if you picked up a handful of mashed potatoes and lobbed it at someone's face as hard as you could.

At best, you'd just really piss this poor person off, but hey, maybe they had it coming!

So what's the difference here?

Why does one form of potato knock someone's teeth out, and the other is what someone's gana have to eat now that they have no teeth?

Cooking breaks down the cellular structure.

The potato is really hard in its uncooked form because, like all plants, it has a rigid cellular structure when raw.

The mashed potatoes are really soft because cooking breaks down the tough membrane that makes the cell rigid.

This is why we get less nutrients from eating raw vegetables.

Our stomach is not capable of cooking our food.

But wouldn't boiling our fresh plant in hot water count as cooking?

For sure, it does, but just like with oil infusions, it has limits to how much it can release, and it has to be boiled the whole time.

Pouring boiling water over a fresh plant would get the process started, but it stops there, and because the plant is already wet, the hot water not only can't be absorbed well into the plant but begins to cool down as soon as you pour it into your jar or cup.

Did you know that drying a plant kinda counts as cooking it?

When we dry a plant, its cellular membranes break down. This is just a natural part of the decaying process.

So when we pour boiling water over the top of dried herbs, a few things happen:

a.) The already weakened and broken down cells release their nutritional values with much more ease than fresh plant matter.

b.) The water is able to saturate the plant's dried-out cells completely, and as it cools, it fully extracts a ton of the nutritional value that we would not get from fresh plant matter.

That is why when you use fresh herbs to try and make any of these things, you are basically just making a very weak broth.

Also, please know I can't be held responsible for any trouble you may get in if you act out the potato experiment half-drunk at some holiday dinner thing you didn't want to go to in the first place.

(With all of that said, if you enjoy making brews with fresh herbs. Go for it!)

8

COLD BREWS

There is this wonderful in-between land of cold brewing herbs that is often overlooked and underutilized.

Here's the catch, though: for the most part, this is really only ideal for fragrant plants where we want these more potent properties vs. nutrients.

Example:

Chamomile is highly fragrant and an amazing friend to work with; we are after her naturally occurring volatile compounds in small amounts, which are what gives her a pleasant aroma. If we were to do a long hot infusion, we would overexact her compounds, making the brew taste horrible and potentially harming you.

VS.

Nettle is a highly nutritious herb with no real fragrant properties, so we are solely after the nutrients. It takes heat and a long brew time to break down the cellular structure and extract these slowly. A quick brewed nettle tea is basically just pointless colored water.

So, with this in mind, cold brews are all about extracting a small amount of the fragrant compounds of a nice-smelling plant without over-extracting a dangerous, nasty-tasting amount of said compounds.

I have actually primarily shifted to making all of my fragrant tea this way so long as I remember to get them started in the evening before bed.

Why?

The flavor is always far more balanced, with a more delicate undertone, and I know that if I am working with a blend, all herbs in the blend have been given the chance to release into the water evenly.

In comparison to a typical cup of hot water tea, where you normally don't want to steep for longer than 10 mins, only the most readily available compound will seep into that water, and we miss out on a lot of benefits while constantly edging over steeping the more potent compounds.

That felt like word salad, but I promise there's a huge difference that's worth experiencing.

9

SUN TEAS

Yet another in-between kinda sorta depends on the brewing method.

When most people think of sun tea, they're from hot summertime climates, and they're probably throwing Liptons or something in a jar with some water, then adding a ton of sugar and calling it sweet tea.

Funnily enough, it is actually made with the true tea plant, not typically herbs.

They're really missing out.

One of my favorite things is making herbal sun tea in the hot months and getting creative!

So, let's talk about how we get away with using fragrant herbs in our sun-heated brew, and this somehow does not over-extract like a tea or hot infusion would.

It's the amount and slow heating.

Because the jar of water and herbs will get blazing hot from the sun, you do not need to put a lot of herbs in there, even if they're not fragrant.

Let's say I'm going to make a lavender lemon sun tea; I'd not add more than 1/4th-½ tsp to a half-gallon jar of water.

Then I'd toss a few sliced lemons in there, maybe some white tea leaves, and call it good come early evening time.

So, when it comes to the fragrant herb I'll be using, it's a very small amount in comparison to the volume of water.

It's like only adding two tiny lavender buds to your cup of tea; there's not enough plant matter to over-extract something on a dangerous level, even if you wanted to.

Then there's the matter of the short infusing time (in comparison to normal herbal infusions) and the fact that, for a good portion of the time, the water is not super hot.

Even where I live in a high mountain desert where we hit 120*F easily, the jar really doesn't get hot to the touch until 3 p.m., and we bring it in around 5, sooner if I'm feeling impatient to try a new creation.

The neat thing about sun teas is because there is heat involved, you can pair nutrient-based herbs like oat straw and fragrant herbs like rose petals.

It's the best of both worlds!

10

TECHNICALLY, IT'S ALL TISANE.

I mean, many people, when they say the word "tea," they're referring to something herbal like chamomile or raspberry vanilla flavored, whatever.

The truth is, though, technically true, tea is only and can only be made from the tea plant Camellia sinensis.

This plant gives us all the classic teas you've likely heard of, like green tea, black tea, white tea, and oolong tea, just to name a few.

The only real differences in true teas come from how the tea leaves are processed and what region they might be grown in.

For example, green tea is less processed, so it stays green; it is typically air-dried or even steamed dry.

On the other hand, black tea is fully oxidized and aged, giving it that dark color.

True teas naturally contain caffeine, whereas herbal teas do not. In fact, not many plants outside of the true tea and coffee bean contain caffeine. It's a pretty rare substance if you think about it.

So, um, if we're not drinking "tea" when we're making herbal tea, what is it?

Technically, it's all tisane.

Literally, if it's made with anything but the Camellia sinensis plant, it's a tisane.

It's all semantics, though; most people just say "herbal tea" vs. "tisane" unless they're trying to sound fancy ha.

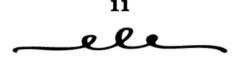

SUPPLIES LIST

Things you will need to get started:

1. A quart-sized canning jar with a lid ½ gallon-sized jars are handy for larger batches.

2. Something to boil water in.

3. Some sort of kitchen scale that can weigh in oz increments.

4. Dried herbs you will be working with.

5. A spoon to stir with.

6. Anything fine mesh to strain with; I prefer nut milk bags or a really tightly woven metal tea strainer.

LET'S MAKE NOURISHING HERBAL INFUSIONS!

Ready for how hard this is gana be?

Weigh out one ounce (28 grams) of your individual dried herb.

Put it in your jar, or better yet, use your jar as the thing you weighed it with. That cuts out the first step.

Bring 4 cups of water to a rolling boil.

Slowly pour the boiling water over the herb.

Once it reaches the top give it a stir, which should make space for you to add a bit more water.

Cap and let it sit for 4-24 hours, placing it in the fridge once it hits room temperature.

After the wait time is up, strain the herb out of the now-infused water.

Your infusion is now ready to drink or use however you intend! Keep them in the fridge and use within three days max for most herbs.

Here are some tips and such:

If you are working with a kinda, slimy plant ally like Comfrey, you may want to consider doing this process twice with the same plant matter.

So after you strain it, you use the herb that you already infused your water with again. This often is when the good, slimy bits that heal mucous membranes are released.

If you are working with someone who has lots of fuzzy hair like Mullein leaf, it's really important that you strain this through a very tightly woven cloth or a mesh nylon nut milk bag. These hairs can often irritate our lungs and stomach lining.

Remember, if a plant has a really strong smell like mint, chamomile, or yarrow, we can't make nourishing herbal infusions out of these because we will extract far too much of their high volatile oil levels.

This can really damage our body and is the same as taking "essential oils" internally.

Plants that are high in proteins, like Stinging Nettle and Oatstraw, usually need to be used up in two days, as they spoil quickly.

When we heal ourselves using nourishment, we need to be patient.

It takes time for these friends to undo the often lifetime of damage we and our situations have done. Give regular use for a solid 3-6 months a chance before you decide it isn't helping you.

Try to cycle through different infusions on a regular basis, and be mindful to know what medicinal actions any one plant has.

Red Clover, for example, is great for hormonal health if you don't have estrogen issues - but she is also a blood thinner and should not be drunk for more than a few days in a row each week.

Don't think you're being clever by putting a bunch of herbs in a jar at once to make an infusion.

Remember this- you will have no idea what plant caused what reaction, whether it's for good or bad if you combine multiple herbs at once.

Also, you shortchange yourself because the one ounce of herb is how much you need of ANY plant to fully saturate the 4 cups of boiling water.

What do we do with the leftover plant matter?

Well, if you're not going to be re-brewing it, you can compost it, feed it to any chickens you may have, or dump it around the base of plants in your garden - or anywhere out on bare earth where it can begin returning to the soil.

Lastly, if you don't have access to any of these places, I'm not gana judge you for putting it in your trashcan like any other food scraps.

Note: Remember nourishing Herbal infusions are like any other food and should be used up in three days.

Yes, you can freeze them if you'd like.

13

LET'S MAKE TEA.

For every person who's like, "I can't believe she just added a section about making tea..this is so basic."

I want you to remember at some point in your life, you had never made tea.

Let alone loose-leaf tea.

Someone reading this book has never made tea, and that's okay, so let's jump right in:

What you'll need:

    1. A teapot or a cup with a lid (for loose-leaf tea).

    2. Loose-leaf herbal tea or tea bags.

3. Boiling water.

4. A strainer (if using loose-leaf tea).

5. A timer (your phone works great).

For Loose Leaf Tea:

1. **Measure it Out:** Use about one Tablespoon of loose-leaf tea per cup of water. If you like it stronger, add a little more; if you prefer it milder, go with less.

2. **Boil Your Water:** Get your water to a rolling boil. Remember, different herbs may need slightly different water temperatures, so don't be afraid to see what Google has to say.

3. **Warm Up the Pot:** If you're using a teapot and want to be fancy about it, pour a bit of boiling water into it and swirl it around to warm it up. Then, pour out the water.

Tip 1: If it's cold in your house, this can prevent your teapot from breaking from thermal shock.

Tip 2: Skip a teapot and just infuse a single cup of tea in your favorite cup using a tea ball or tea infuser of some variety.

1. **Brew Time:** Add your tea leaves to the teapot or directly into your cup. Pour in the hot water.

2. **Time It:** Start the timer and let the tea steep. Most herbal teas need about 8-10 minutes, but some might need longer. Typically, if it's a root, it needs longer; if it's fragrant, don't go much past 10 minutes.

3. Strain and Sip: When the timer goes off, pour the tea through a strainer into your cup if you're using a teapot. If you're using a cup with a lid, just remove the lid and pull out whatever you used to infuse your tea with.

For Pre-Made Tea Bags:

1. **Water Boiling Time:** Boil some water. Yep, same as

before.

2. **Tea Bag in a Mug:** Pop your tea bag into a mug.

Tip: There's not much in a store-bought tea bag; if I use these, I typically add 2-4 tea bags per cup because I want it to be beneficial, not just colored water.

1. **Pour Hot Water:** Pour the boiling water over the tea bag.

2. **Cover and Steep:** Cover your mug with a small plate, canning jar lid, whatever, just anything that'll keep the heat in. Let it steep for the recommended time on the packaging, usually 3-8 minutes.

3. **Remove and Enjoy:** After the steeping time is up, take out the tea bag and **resist** squeezing it against the side of the mug; this can make it bitter.

Remember, everyone's taste is different, so feel free to experiment with tea strength and steeping times until you find your perfect cup. And don't be afraid to add honey, sugar, lemon, or even a splash of milk!

14

LET'S MAKE A COLD BREW.

We're about to unlock the secret to preserving all those aromatic and delicate flavors from your choice of fragrant herbs without over-extracting them in hot water.

It's absurdly easy.

Ingredients:

1. Highly scented herbs (like lavender, mint, or chamomile).

2. Cold water.

3. A glass container or mason jar.

4. A fine-mesh strainer or tea filter.

5. Time and patience.

Step 1: Herb Selection

First things first, choose your highly scented herbs.

I keep saying "highly scented" because this really won't work well with herbs that are not fragrant.

You can get creative with combinations, but no matter what, it's important to select herbs that have fragrance.

Consider classics like lavender, mint, chamomile, or rose petals.

I really love chamomile paired with a sprinkling of lavender buds; I have a fresh jar of this brewing darn near nightly just waiting for me in the morning.

Tip: If it smells bitter or pungent as a fragrance (like valerian root), your brew will taste like it smells. Proceed with knowledge.

Step 2: Measure Your Herbs

For a standard quart jar (4 cups water) container, you'll want about 1/4th - ½ cups of your chosen herbs.

Tip: I suggest starting at the ¼ cup mark and working your way up; it is better to need more herbs and drink a weaker brew than to go too strong and dump out what you have made because it's too strong to drink.

Step 3: Actually making it.

Place your herbs in a glass container or mason jar. Pour cold water over the herbs.

Now, put a cap on whatever you're using to infuse and give it a good shake.

As an FYI, you could not do this with hot water; it would spray out of the cap and burn you.

This is where the magic of cold brewing happens. By using cold water, you're not shocking the herbs with high temperatures, which can over-extract and, in some ways, under-extract their fragrant properties at the same weird time.

Step 5: Infuse and Wait

Now, the easiest part – waiting!

Let your herbal concoction sit in your fridge for about 8-10 hours.

This is why I always start my cold brews just before I go to bed and strain them in the morning.

This slow extraction process lets the herbs release their scent and flavor without being forced by hot water. The volatile oils in the herbs stay in balance, giving you a wonderfully aromatic tea.

Step 6: Strain and Serve

Once your brew has had its beauty steep (cheap puns are great, ha), it's time to strain it.

Use a fine-mesh strainer or a tea filter to catch all the herb bits, leaving you with a clear, fragrant liquid.

From here, you can drink it over ice or simply warm up a cup's worth if you want a warm tea.

With my favorite chamomile and lavender blend, I typically add a bit of sugar and a splash of raw goat milk (thank you, Martha and Betty, my milk goats), poured over ice; even in the winter time, this is typically the first thing I drink in the morning.

These cold brews are usually good for about three days in the fridge, so if you find a blend you like or have a fragrant herb you really want to work with on a daily basis, don't be afraid to make a half gallon at a time so you only have to make a new one every three days or so. It's super handy!

15

LET'S MAKE SUN TEA.

This is the most creative option out of all the types I have covered, so feel free to go wild here and have fun thinking of new sun tea recipes!

1. Gather Your Supplies

First things first, you'll need some loose-leaf herbal tea. Choose your favorite flavor; it could be something soothing like chamomile or a cooling mix of peppermint and lemon verbena.

You'll also need a glass jar with a lid or a pitcher, water, and some fruit (fresh or dry works) to make something truly amazing.

Lemons, berries, and peaches work great.

2. Fill Your Container

Get your jar or pitcher and fill it with water. Go for about 4 cups (or 1 liter/quart) of water. Starting from cold works best.

3. Add Your Herbs

Now comes the fun part. Take 1/4th cup-½ cup MAX of loose-leaf herbal tea (adjust to your taste) and drop them into the water.

If you're using a jar, give it a good stir so the tea leaves don't hang out kinda dry at the top. Put the lid on.

4. Sweeten It Up (Optional)

If you like your tea sweet, this is when you can add a little honey or sugar to your jar before you place it in the sun. Stir it in and adjust to your taste.

Some folks "freak out" thinking the sugar setting for that long will make the tea "sour" from bacteria and say to add it at the end.

Ironically, the lack of sugar in the water can actually be why bacteria can grow. It's why we can water bath can things like fruit (high sugar) and make them shelf stable and why we have to use a pressure cooker for low sugar things such as vegetables (no sugar).

Sugar inhibits bacterial growth.

Honestly, though, it's a) not setting out there long enough to go bad, and b) it gets really hot from the sun, killing off anything that tried to grow.

I just like to add my sugar before infusing because, honestly, it mixes in better and is easier.

5. **Let the Sun Shine On It.**

Place your jar or pitcher in a sunny spot in the **direct** sun.

A table, porch, or anywhere outside where the jar will get sun for most, if not all, of the day.

The heat of the sun will infuse your tea with flavor.

Most folks will tell you to leave it for a few hours, usually 2-4, depending on how strong you want it.

I, however, typically put mine out by 10 a.m. and pull it in around 4 p.m., so I shoot for 6-7 hours!

6. Strain

When your sun tea brew time is up, it's time to strain it.

If you've added fruit directly to the tea, you'll want to kinda give it a good squeeze after straining to get the juice out. I will say it's best not to leave the fruit in for drinking as it will make the sun tea go off fast in the fridge, and they'll be kinda slimy and not something you really want floating in your cup. It's cooked fruit.

7. Chill and Enjoy

Let your tea cool down a bit on the counter, like lukewarm, then pop it into the fridge to cool it down all the way, or pour it over ice.

Feel free to get creative with your fruit choices and experiment with different herbs.

Tip: Write down your experiments because it's a bummer to make an awesome sun tea and not be able to re-create it fully!

Here are some great blends to try:

Citrus Mint Sun Tea:

2 TBSP mint leaf

1 lemon, sliced

1 orange, sliced

4 cups of water

Strawberry Basil Sun Tea:

4 TBSP white tea

1 cup fresh strawberries, sliced

3 fresh basil leaves

4 cups of water

Pineapple Ginger Sun Tea:

2 TBSP freshly grated ginger root

1 cup fresh pineapple chunks, canned will not work as well here.

4 cups of water

Blueberry Thyme Sun Tea:

1 healthy sprig of fresh thyme; dry won't work well.

2 cups fresh or frozen blueberries

4 cups of water

16

HOW TO BLEND TEAS AT HOME

Blending your own herbal teas at home can seem intimidating, but they're actually pretty easy and a fun way to build a relationship with herbs.

While this can be a never-ending deep dive subject in the realms of herbalism, I'm going to do my best to explain this in a simple way because too much complexity is what typically stops folks from trying!

So here's a step-by-step guide on how to get started with literally zero experience needed:

First, let's talk Materials and Tools:

Dried herbs:

You can purchase these from just about anywhere online (Google+the herb you want to buy), dry your own herbs from your garden, or wildcraft them from your local area.

Airtight containers:

For storing your ingredients and finished tea blends. For long-term storage, I highly suggest vacuum seal bags or jars.

If you make a lot of tea, glass jars are a pain, take up a lot of space, and tend to break.

When I vacuum seal herbs, I can toss them in my freezer or a big storage tote and don't have to worry about them breaking or taking up valuable cupboard space.

Mixing bowls or jars:

For blending and storing.

Technically, it's called "garbling" when you mix herbs together, especially if you are plucking leaves or removing stems, but I often feel that "specialist" words like that make people feel...pushed out.

It's mixing. Just call it mixing.

A tea infuser or a teapot with an infuser basket.

Kitchen scale:

If you *truly* want to recreate anything you end up loving, you absolutely need to write down your ingredients by weight.

If you can't swing a kitchen scale, at the very least, use cup measurements so you can get close to recreating what you have made.

Labels/Notebook:

To keep track of your blends. Write down everything you do, no matter how small; it matters.

Okay, first, I'm going to help you *think* about how a tea blend is made in sections that will make up a whole, then give you some visual-spatial examples because that's just how my brain works.

Base Herbs:

In human speak, this means it's the *largest* amount of an herb used in your formula, and more often than not, a base herb is a non-fragrant one, so you can use a lot of it without being overwhelmed by the flavor.

A few good examples would be oat straw, raspberry leaf, nettle, and rooibos.

It's not that these herbs don't have a flavor. It's that they don't have a strong fragrance, which allows us to layer flavors over the top with fragrant herbs without making too potent of a blend.

Flavor Enhancers:

These herbs add depth and complexity to your tea blends & are typically used in smaller amounts.

Things like lavender, lemongrass, rose, cinnamon, or citrus peels are good examples of flavor enhancers.

We want to use smaller amounts of fragrant herbs due to the higher volatile compounds that are easily over-brewed, easily bitter, or too strong, so a little goes a long way.

Functional Herbs:

This is always kind of a weird category to me because all herbs are functional; they all do something for or to our bodies.

In the realms of tea making, though, functional herbs tend to mean one of or all of the following:

a.) The herb that delivers the primary desired action.

b.) A pungent herb that does not have the best flavor.

c.) A powerful herb that needs to be used in small amounts.

It could be that your base herb is your functional herb; it is easy to overthink this, I know.

Here comes the visual-spatial:

When you make a recipe, any recipe, there are big amounts of ingredients and small amounts of ingredients.

The largest amount of something is the "base" of the entire thing.

Everything after that is either a *flavor enhancer* or something *functional*.

Example:

Let's make some cookies!

Flour in your chocolate chip cookies would be the base ingredient.

Vanilla, salt, and chocolate chips in your cookies would be *flavor-enhancing* ingredients.

The baking powder would be a *functional* ingredient, so the cookies rise a bit.

I know we're making an herbal tea blend, not tasty cookies, but I promise getting you to think in layers and how something works in a blend is super helpful.

Once I get your brain to think in layers, you can make up tea blends on the spot like this one I'm literally making up as I type this:

We'll call it "April's sleepy tea."

Base herb: Oat Straw 4 cups.

Flavor enhance herb: Chamomile 1 cup.

Functional herb: Skullcap ¼ cup.

The oat straw has a very mild flavor but is a good one for the nervous system, so we can use this as the bulk of the tea.

The chamomile has a distinct flavor, of course, and is well-known as a relaxing herb.

Skullcap doesn't taste bad but is potent; even though a lot of her sedative properties dissipate once dried, she still needs to be used in smaller amounts, or we can feel nauseated/spinny vs. sleepy.

So, all of the herbs in this blend would support a good night's sleep and stress reduction, but we go from gentle to potent, slowly lowering the amounts from base to flavoring to functional.

From here, you have got to start tasting and *feeling* your tea to begin making adjustments.

Tip: If you want your flavor-enhancing herbs to be more forward-tasting in your blend, scale back on your base herb vs. increasing your flavor-enhancing herb.

This often results in a more balanced flavor where you don't wash out your base layer taste yet bring out more of the flavor-enhancing herb.

Let's look at an example:

You are thinking of adding an additional ½ cup of chamomile for a more forward flavor because the oat straw is too strong and washing out the chamomile flavor.

Instead of adding more chamomile, add ½ cup **less of the base herb** oat straw in your next blending.

The chamomile will naturally be more forward as you scale back the base herb because there is now more chamomile in every scoop of tea you are brewing because there is *less* oat straw.

This is also cost-effective because fragrant herbs are often more expensive than non-fragrant herbs, which are what typically make up our base herb.

So what if you feel like the skullcap is too strong or not strong enough?

Of course, you can always scale back, but if you feel like your flavor is close to spot on, it's yet again best to adjust the base layer instead of the functional herb.

So, instead of cutting back or increasing the skullcap, slightly increase or decrease the base herb, oat straw.

I want you to look at your base herb as a dial to be turned up or down to increase or decrease the taste or actions of your flavor or functional herb.

Okay, so you are thinking in layers and now know the key to all of this is adjusting your base herb and want to give it a go?

Here are a few questions that will help you figure out what herbs to use:

What do you want your tea to "do." ?

Looking for digestive support? Need to get some sleep? Immune support? Relaxation?

This question is the most important because this is how you will pick out your core herb(s) in the blend, and it will likely influence everything else.

You'll notice in my theoretical "April's Sleepy Tea" blend that I combined herbs that all have similar action(s) like sleep, relaxation, and nervous system support.

You will want to do the same or find herbs that complement one another.

I know it can feel overwhelming to research herbs, but let me give you a place to start:

"Google_____What gentle herbs are good for XYZ issue."

From here, you will likely see a plethora of herbs that all have similar actions, and you can begin looking into each herb and then decide who may go well with one another and your personal needs.

I know folks will scoff at me for saying to use a search engine, but why? The internet literally holds all information, and you are smart enough to read and make decisions no matter what anyone tells you!

Next question:

What herb will you use to help your tea "do" what you're wanting, and is this herb fragrant or not?

If the herb is **not fragrant**, this will likely become your *entire* **base** herb.

If the herb **is fragrant**, consider making this either your **functional herb** or your **flavor enhancer**.

Really, when looking to make a tea blend, there are no rules to how many herbs you add to a blend, but 2-4 is typically the sweet spot.

Anything more than four herbs becomes...a little more complex, and you will want to make very small sample blends and do constant taste testing.

Which you can absolutely do complicated!

I know you can!

Yet, if you start simple, working your way up to more complex blends will give you a beautiful foundation for understanding herbal tea blending.

For the analytical folks in the crowd, let's talk ratios:

Beginners can start by using a simple ratio for their base layer.

A typical ratio for a base layer is 2 parts of the primary base herb, 1 part of the secondary flavor-enhancing herb, and ½ part of the functional herb.

For example, if you're creating a blend for digestion, you might use 2 parts chamomile, 1 part spearmint, and ½ part ginger root.

Whatever you do, and however you do it...write it all down!

Mixing Your Blend

You can use a big bowl to mix in; you can put all of your herbs in a jar and shake, or you can set the herbs in a ziplock bag and shake the heck out of it!

There really is no wrong way to mix something together, although I feel like I need to say... probably don't use a food processor.

The beauty of blending your own herbal teas is that you can experiment endlessly.

Try different combinations, ratios, and ingredients to find the flavor and health support you love and need the most.

In no time at all, you'll become skilled at crafting your own herbal tea creations that you & your loved ones will be happy to have on hand.

17

COMMON HERBS USED FOR NOURISHING HERBAL INFUSIONS

There are so many herbs that can be used as nourishing herbal infusions. It's just important to remember that **fragrant herbs should not be used** for long brewed infusions, and of course, the herb needs to be edible.

Below, I'll give a rundown of the most common herbs used with nourishing herbal infusions.

Nettle (Urtica dioica):

1 oz per quart jar

Common Names: Nettle, Stinging Nettle.

Vitamin Content: Nettle is a rich source of vitamins, particularly vitamin A, vitamin C, vitamin K, and several B vitamins. It's also high in minerals such as iron, calcium, and magnesium.

Healing Compounds: Nettle contains flavonoids, carotenoids, and chlorophyll, which contribute to her health benefits. She's also known for her high content of iron and other nutrients.

Health Benefits: Nettle is prized for her nourishing and tonic properties.

She is known to support the immune system, thyroid, and adrenal, promote healthy skin, and aid detoxification through the lymphatic pathways.

Nettle infusions are often used to alleviate allergies, support the circulatory system, and improve energy. I love her for chronic fatigue.

Additionally, nettle is commonly used as a natural remedy for joint pain and arthritis, and many folks even seek out fresh nettle in the spring to sting themselves on sore joints for arthritis relief.

Cautions: Nettle is generally safe when used as a nourishing infusion or food, but fresh, she can cause skin irritation due to her "stinging" hairs that actually fling a tiny drop of acid that causes a histamine reaction.

There is no risk of sting from dried nettle.

Medications/Conditions to Consider: Nettle may interact with anticoagulant drugs, blood pressure medications, and diuretics. Anyone with a history of kidney stones or those taking lithium should use Nettle cautiously due to her diuretic effect.

Oat Straw (Avena sativa):

1 oz per quart jar

Common Names: Oat Straw, Oat Tops.

Vitamin Content: Oat straw is a good source of vitamins, including vitamin B1 (thiamine), vitamin B2 (riboflavin), and vitamin E.

Healing Compounds: The healing compounds in oat straw include saponins, flavonoids, and minerals such as silica, calcium, and magnesium.

Health Benefits: Oat straw infusions are known for their calming and nerve-soothing properties, and I love her for long-term stress support. They are often used to relieve stress, anxiety, and nervous tension. Oat straw is also great for healthy skin, supports the skeletal system, and enhances digestion.

Then there's the lowering of cholesterol and heart health; basically, every healthy thing you have heard about oatmeal should be applied to oat straw because oat straw is made from the stems of oats. The plant that we get oats/oatmeal from!

Cautions: Oat straw is considered safe when used appropriately, but allergies to oats can occur, and **it's crucial** to source organic as conventional oats are a really dirty crop heavy with pesticides.

Medications/Conditions to Consider: There are generally no known interactions or contraindications with medications or conditions related to oat straw consumption; I mean, it's oatmeal...

However, anyone with gluten sensitivities should ensure they use gluten-free oat straw so the equipment used to harvest is not contaminated with previous wheat crops.

Linden Blooms (Tilia spp.):

½ oz per quart jar can be infused 2x.

Common Names: Linden Blossoms, Lime Flowers.

Vitamin Content: Linden blooms are not exceptionally high in vitamins, but they contain trace amounts of vitamin C and other antioxidants.

Healing Compounds: The main healing compounds in linden blossoms are flavonoids, mucilage, and trace amounts of volatile oils such as Farnesene, Citral, Nerol, and Linalool.

Note: This is the only vaguely fragrant herb I will make a nourishing herbal infusion from because her VOC levels are really low.

Health Benefits: Linden infusions are renowned for their calming and soothing effects. They are often used as a remedy for anxiety, insomnia, and stress. Linden is gentle on the digestive system and can provide relief from indigestion and upset stomach.

She is also known for her mild diaphoretic properties, which in human words means she opens up your pores so heat can escape, which helps alleviate fever and support the immune system.

She is also fantastic for cardiovascular support, and I really think she shines for people who are so burnt out from stressors that their immune system has begun to suffer.

She is also gentle enough that herbalists for hundreds of years have used her for children with colds and fevers.

Cautions: Linden is considered safe in moderation, but excessive consumption may lead to heart-related side effects. I'm talking don't drink a gallon a day...

Medications/Conditions to Consider: Avoid linden if you are taking medications that affect the heart, as linden can enhance the effects of these drugs. If you have heart conditions, consult your healthcare provider before using linden infusions.

Red Clover (Trifolium pratense):

1 oz per quart jar

Common Names: Red Clover

Vitamin Content: Red clover is a good source of vitamins such as C, B1 (thiamine), B3 (niacin).

Healing Compounds: Red clover contains isoflavones, coumarins, and flavonoids.

Health Benefits: Red clover infusions are often used to support hormonal balance, especially in women. They can alleviate menopausal symptoms and PMS, especially heavy cramping.

Red clover is also known for her blood-cleansing properties and can improve skin conditions like acne. Additionally, she can help boost the immune system and reduce inflammation with her slight blood thinning properties.

Lastly, she is renowned for her fertility-increasing abilities and has helped many women to conceive.

Cautions: Red clover is generally safe when used in moderation, but it may cause minor side effects like headaches or nausea in some.

Because she is a blood thinner, it's important to take breaks from her and consider working with a Vitamin K supplement if you will be using her long-term to combat the blood thinning effects.

Medications/Conditions to Consider: Red clover will interact with blood-thinning medications and hormone-related drugs. She should be avoided if you have a history of hormone-related conditions like breast cancer or uterine fibroids due to her phytoestrogen content.

Mallow Root (Malva spp.):

1 oz per quart jar/ can be made with cold water.

Common Names: Mallow Root, Button Weed, Cheese Plant.

Vitamin Content: Mallow root contains vitamins A and C.

Healing Compounds: Mallow root is rich in mucilage, which gives it soothing and demulcent properties alongside flavonoids and anthocyanidins.

Health Benefits: Mallow root infusions are often used to alleviate inflammation and irritation in the respiratory and digestive tracts. If you have leaky gut or something like G. E.R.D, you need mallow in your life!

She can soothe coughs, sore throats, and digestive discomfort. Mallow root is also beneficial for skin health and can be used topically to treat skin conditions; I love her for all things poison oak/ivy etc.. Additionally, she supports healthy mucous membranes from mouth to rear!

Cautions: Mallow root is generally safe, but in rare cases, it may cause allergic reactions.

Medications/Conditions to Consider: There are no specific known interactions or contraindications with medications or conditions related to mallow root. However, if you experience an allergic reaction, discontinue use.

Plantain Leaf (Plantago major):

Common Names: Plantain Leaf, Broadleaf Plantain, White Mans Foot.

Vitamin Content: Plantain leaf contains vitamins A and C.

Healing Compounds: Plantain leaf is rich in mucilage, tannins, and allantoin.

Health Benefits: Plantain leaf infusions are known for their soothing and healing properties. They can be used to alleviate respiratory issues, including coughs and congestion.

Plantain is also applied topically to promote wound healing and relieve skin irritations like insect bites and rashes; you can drink the infusion and use the leftover infused plant matter to make a topical poultice!

She supports the health of mucous membranes and can be beneficial for respiratory and digestive health.

One of her main compounds, allantoin, is the same property in comfrey that stimulates new cell development and bone healing. So, she is a great alternative for those who may be nervous about using Comfrey internally.

Cautions: Plantain leaf is considered safe as a nourishing herb, but she can cause skin allergies in some individuals.

Medications/Conditions to Consider: There are generally no known interactions or contraindications with medications or conditions related to plantain leaf consumption. However, if you experience skin irritation or allergies, discontinue use.

Including nourishing herbal infusions into your daily routine can drastically change your health for the better as we deeply renourish our body, knock down inflammation, heal our guts, and boost our immune system.

I would be far closer to death (kidding, not kidding) if it weren't for nourishing herbal infusions!

They are pretty affordable too, if you look at how much liquid you end up getting.

There are 16 ounces in a pound; it's typically 1 oz per 4 cups (quart) of water.

This means with a single pound of herb, you can make four gallons worth of infusion to drink.

Most people don't typically drink more than a quart of infusion daily.

18

MAKE SURE TO CHANGE THINGS UP!

I know I have talked about this a bit already, but let's dig a little bit deeper to really drive it home.

Cycling through nourishing herbal infusions and teas is a really smart way to keep from getting burnt out and have the highest chance of restoring your health.

Let's jabber about why it's important:

Variety is the Spice of Life: Like with food, a varied diet is vital. Different herbs provide a wide range of nutrients, and cycling through them ensures you get a diverse set of vitamins, minerals, and phytonutrients.

Prevent Sensitivities: Overusing the same herb can lead to sensitivities or allergies. By switching it up, you reduce the risk of your body becoming too accustomed to any one herb, causing weird things to happen.

Avoid Overloading: Herbs have real effects on the body. Cycling through various herbs gives your system a break from the impacts. Even if they are beneficial, they can become a stressor.

Build a Relationship with Many Herbs: There's a whole world of herbs out there, each with unique benefits. Cycling through them lets you explore this herbal diversity, learning which ones work best for your body and individual needs. Herbs are not one size fits all!

Prevent Routine Burnout: Just as you can get stuck in a food rut, drinking the same tea or infusion every day can become boring. By mixing it up, you keep your herbal routine exciting and enjoyable.

Mind-Body Connection: Switching herbs can be a mindful practice, helping you connect with your body's changing needs and your evolving relationship with herbs.

The 3-Day Herbal Infusion Cycle:

Day 1-3: Nettle (Urtica dioica):

Nettle offers a rich source of vitamins and minerals, making her an excellent choice to start your cycle.

Her energy-boosting properties are a great way to kick things off.

Day 4-6: Linden Blossoms (Tilia spp.):

Linden provides a calming and soothing experience. She's ideal for those looking to unwind and reduce stress.

Enjoy her mild, floral flavor during this phase of the cycle.

Day 7-9: Mallow Root (Malva spp.):

Mallow root can help soothe your digestive and respiratory systems.

She's a great herb to introduce after linden to provide additional/consistent relief from potential gut issues.

Day 10-12: Oat Straw (Avena sativa):

Oat straw is known for her calming and nerve-soothing properties, which is beneficial for your probably stressed-out body.

It's a great addition after mallow root to keep your gut calm by targeting the nervous system with a calcium boost.

Day 13-15: Plantain Leaf (Plantago major):

Plantain leaf will literally trigger your body to produce new cells and begin healing various issues.

Look at what I did with this lineup, in case you missed it:

Day 1-3 I deeply nourished my thyroid/adrenals & supported my kidney functions.

Day 4-9 I targeted gut health to calm stress hormones and support immune functions.

Day 10-12 I targeted the nervous system, saying, "We are safe, we can rest," with the needed calcium to do so,

Day 13-15 I said okay, now let's make some new cells, heal some issues, and use the momentum we have built up to make a real difference.

Repeat the Cycle: Once you've completed the 15-day cycle, start over and complete the month.

Most people see real change in the first three months and will become lifelong advocates of nourishing herbal infusions by the time they are an entirely new person in six months to a year!

So get yourself some herbs, some jars, and boil up some water because great things are about to happen for your health as soon as you get started!

19

IN CONCLUSION

Despite many other herbalists insisting that you need to study for hours, days, weeks, months, or years before you can make your own tea blends, be "smart enough" to work with infusions, or anything else, nourishing herbal infusions and teas of any kind are a beautiful way to begin practicing herbalism.

When we choose to work with safe, humble plants, it is exceptionally hard to truly hurt ourselves or others in any lasting way, especially if we stick to nourishing-based herbs and take our time to get to know which herbs we will be working with.

They get us curious about what might be growing in our own backyard; they make us seek out nature, our local farms, and the community at large, and online resources as we look for plants we are pulled to work with.

They can be highly affordable when you buy herbs in bulk, especially when you compare the cost to buying things like ready-made tea or expensive, less nourishing juices.

Most importantly, you are absolutely smart enough to do this!

20

KEEP LEARNING

Common Ways For Common People - Volume One - Tinctures & Elixirs - April Graham

Common Ways For Common People - Volume Two - Herbal Infused Oils - April Graham

Common Ways For Common People - Volume Three- Balms, Salves, Butters - April Graham

Essentially Deadly: The Unspoken Dangers Of Essential Oils - April Graham

Getting Started With Compliance - Record-Keeping - April Graham

Spare Changing For Trauma - A memoir of pain and healing
- April Graham.

www.youtube.com/@sheisofthewoods 200+ Free simple
herbal how-to videos - April Graham

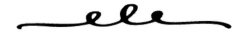

PERSONAL NOTES

In this section, you can keep track of the little things you notice, like:

Did one batch of tea turn out tastier than another even though it's the same ingredient?

What did you do differently? Did you harvest the herbs or buy them?

Did you like the sun tea version better tea? Did you try it both ways?

How long did a certain batch of blended tea last you?

Did you discover something new?

Something helpful? Did you figure something out?

As we keep track of subtle things, we learn the small nuances that make big differences in quality over years of teas & infusions, so please know nothing is so small it's not worth writing down!

Notes About:_____ Date: _/_/_

_____
_____
_____
_____

Notes About:_____ Date: _/_/_

_____
_____
_____
_____

Notes About:_____ Date: _/_/_

_____
_____
_____
_____

Notes About:_____ Date: _/_/_

_____
_____
_____
_____

Notes About:_____ Date: __/__/__

_____

_____

_____

_____

Notes About:_____ Date: __/__/__

_____

_____

_____

_____

Notes About:_____ Date: __/__/__

_____

_____

_____

_____

Notes About:_____ Date: __/__/__

_____

_____

_____

_____

Notes About:_____ Date: __/__/__

_____
_____
_____
_____

Notes About:_____ Date: __/__/__

_____
_____
_____
_____

Notes About:_____ Date: __/__/__

_____
_____
_____
_____

Notes About:_____ Date: __/__/__

_____
_____
_____
_____

Notes About:_____ Date: _/_/_

_____
_____
_____
_____

Notes About:_____ Date: _/_/_

_____
_____
_____
_____

Notes About:_____ Date: _/_/_

_____
_____
_____
_____

Notes About:_____ Date: _/_/_

_____
_____
_____
_____

Notes About:_____ Date: __/__/__

_____

_____

_____

_____

Notes About:_____ Date: __/__/__

_____

_____

_____

_____

Notes About:_____ Date: __/__/__

_____

_____

_____

_____

Notes About:_____ Date: __/__/__

_____

_____

_____

_____

Notes About:_____ Date: _/_/_

_____
_____
_____
_____

Notes About:_____ Date: _/_/_

_____
_____
_____
_____

Notes About:_____ Date: _/_/_

_____
_____
_____
_____

Notes About:_____ Date: _/_/_

_____
_____
_____
_____

Notes About:_____ Date: __/__/__

_____
_____
_____
_____

Notes About:_____ Date: __/__/__

_____
_____
_____
_____

Notes About:_____ Date: __/__/__

_____
_____
_____
_____

Notes About:_____ Date: __/__/__

_____
_____
_____
_____

Notes About:_____ Date: __/__/__

_____
_____
_____
_____

Notes About:_____ Date: __/__/__

_____
_____
_____
_____

Notes About:_____ Date: __/__/__

_____
_____
_____
_____

Notes About:_____ Date: __/__/__

_____
_____
_____
_____

Notes About:_____ Date: __/__/__

_____

_____

_____

_____

Notes About:_____ Date: __/__/__

_____

_____

_____

_____

Notes About:_____ Date: __/__/__

_____

_____

_____

_____

Notes About:_____ Date: __/__/__

_____

_____

_____

_____

Notes About:_____ Date: _/_/_

_____
_____
_____
_____

Notes About:_____ Date: _/_/_

_____
_____
_____
_____

Notes About:_____ Date: _/_/_

_____
_____
_____
_____

Notes About:_____ Date: _/_/_

_____
_____
_____
_____

Notes About:_____ Date: _/_/_

_____
_____
_____
_____

Notes About:_____ Date: _/_/_

_____
_____
_____
_____

Notes About:_____ Date: _/_/_

_____
_____
_____
_____

Notes About:_____ Date: _/_/_

_____
_____
_____
_____

Notes About:_____ Date: _/_/_

_____
_____
_____
_____

Notes About:_____ Date: _/_/_

_____
_____
_____
_____

Notes About:_____ Date: _/_/_

_____
_____
_____
_____

Notes About:_____ Date: _/_/_

_____
_____
_____
_____

Notes About:_____ Date: __/__/__

_____
_____
_____
_____

Notes About:_____ Date: __/__/__

_____
_____
_____
_____

Notes About:_____ Date: __/__/__

_____
_____
_____
_____

Notes About:_____ Date: __/__/__

_____
_____
_____
_____

Notes About:_____ Date: _/_/_

_____
_____
_____
_____

Notes About:_____ Date: _/_/_

_____
_____
_____
_____

Notes About:_____ Date: _/_/_

_____
_____
_____
_____

Notes About:_____ Date: _/_/_

_____
_____
_____
_____

Notes About:_____ Date: _/_/_

_____
_____
_____
_____

Notes About:_____ Date: _/_/_

_____
_____
_____
_____

Notes About:_____ Date: _/_/_

_____
_____
_____
_____

Notes About:_____ Date: _/_/_

_____
_____
_____
_____

Notes About:_____ Date: _/_/_

_____
_____
_____
_____

Notes About:_____ Date: _/_/_

_____
_____
_____
_____

Notes About:_____ Date: _/_/_

_____
_____
_____
_____

Notes About:_____ Date: _/_/_

_____
_____
_____
_____

Notes About:_____ Date: _/_/_

_____
_____
_____
_____

Notes About:_____ Date: _/_/_

_____
_____
_____
_____

Notes About:_____ Date: _/_/_

_____
_____
_____
_____

Notes About:_____ Date: _/_/_

_____
_____
_____
_____

Notes About:_____ Date: __/__/__

_____

_____

_____

_____

Notes About:_____ Date: __/__/__

_____

_____

_____

_____

Notes About:_____ Date: __/__/__

_____

_____

_____

_____

Notes About:_____ Date: __/__/__

_____

_____

_____

_____

Notes About:_____ Date: _/_/_

_____
_____
_____
_____

Notes About:_____ Date: _/_/_

_____
_____
_____
_____

Notes About:_____ Date: _/_/_

_____
_____
_____
_____

Notes About:_____ Date: _/_/_

_____
_____
_____
_____

Notes About:_____ Date: _/_/_

_____
_____
_____
_____

Notes About:_____ Date: _/_/_

_____
_____
_____
_____

Notes About:_____ Date: _/_/_

_____
_____
_____
_____

Notes About:_____ Date: _/_/_

_____
_____
_____
_____

Notes About:_____ Date: __/__/__

_____

_____

_____

_____

Notes About:_____ Date: __/__/__

_____

_____

_____

_____

Notes About:_____ Date: __/__/__

_____

_____

_____

_____

Notes About:_____ Date: __/__/__

_____

_____

_____

_____

Notes About:_____ Date: _/_/_

_____
_____
_____
_____

Notes About:_____ Date: _/_/_

_____
_____
_____
_____

Notes About:_____ Date: _/_/_

_____
_____
_____
_____

Notes About:_____ Date: _/_/_

_____
_____
_____
_____

Notes About:_____ Date: _/_/_

_____
_____
_____
_____

Notes About:_____ Date: _/_/_

_____
_____
_____
_____

Notes About:_____ Date: _/_/_

_____
_____
_____
_____

Notes About:_____ Date: _/_/_

_____
_____
_____
_____

Notes About:_____ Date: __/__/__

_____
_____
_____
_____

Notes About:_____ Date: __/__/__

_____
_____
_____
_____

Notes About:_____ Date: __/__/__

_____
_____
_____
_____

Notes About:_____ Date: __/__/__

_____
_____
_____
_____

Notes About:_____ Date: __/__/__

_____

_____

_____

_____

Notes About:_____ Date: __/__/__

_____

_____

_____

_____

Notes About:_____ Date: __/__/__

_____

_____

_____

_____

Notes About:_____ Date: __/__/__

_____

_____

_____

_____

Notes About:_____ Date: _/_/_

_____

_____

_____

_____

Notes About:_____ Date: _/_/_

_____

_____

_____

_____

Notes About:_____ Date: _/_/_

_____

_____

_____

_____

Notes About:_____ Date: _/_/_

_____

_____

_____

_____

Notes About:_____ Date: __/__/__

_____
_____
_____
_____

Notes About:_____ Date: __/__/__

_____
_____
_____
_____

Notes About:_____ Date: __/__/__

_____
_____
_____
_____

Notes About:_____ Date: __/__/__

_____
_____
_____
_____

Notes About:_____ Date: __/__/__

_____
_____
_____
_____

Notes About:_____ Date: __/__/__

_____
_____
_____
_____

Notes About:_____ Date: __/__/__

_____
_____
_____
_____

Notes About:_____ Date: __/__/__

_____
_____
_____
_____

Notes About:_____ Date: __/__/__

_____
_____
_____
_____

Notes About:_____ Date: __/__/__

_____
_____
_____
_____

Notes About:_____ Date: __/__/__

_____
_____
_____
_____

Notes About:_____ Date: __/__/__

_____
_____
_____
_____

Notes About:_____ Date: _/_/_

_____

_____

_____

_____

Notes About:_____ Date: _/_/_

_____

_____

_____

_____

Notes About:_____ Date: _/_/_

_____

_____

_____

_____

Notes About:_____ Date: _/_/_

_____

_____

_____

_____

Notes About:_____ Date: __/__/__

_____
_____
_____
_____

Notes About:_____ Date: __/__/__

_____
_____
_____
_____

Notes About:_____ Date: __/__/__

_____
_____
_____
_____

Notes About:_____ Date: __/__/__

_____
_____
_____
_____

Notes About:_____ Date: __/__/__

_____
_____
_____
_____

Notes About:_____ Date: __/__/__

_____
_____
_____
_____

Notes About:_____ Date: __/__/__

_____
_____
_____
_____

Notes About:_____ Date: __/__/__

_____
_____
_____
_____

Notes About:_____ Date: _/_/_

_____
_____
_____
_____

Notes About:_____ Date: _/_/_

_____
_____
_____
_____

Notes About:_____ Date: _/_/_

_____
_____
_____
_____

Notes About:_____ Date: _/_/_

_____
_____
_____
_____

Notes About:_____ Date: _/_/_

_____
_____
_____
_____

Notes About:_____ Date: _/_/_

_____
_____
_____
_____

Notes About:_____ Date: _/_/_

_____
_____
_____
_____

Notes About:_____ Date: _/_/_

_____
_____
_____
_____

Notes About:_____ Date: __/__/__

_____
_____
_____
_____

Notes About:_____ Date: __/__/__

_____
_____
_____
_____

Notes About:_____ Date: __/__/__

_____
_____
_____
_____

Notes About:_____ Date: __/__/__

_____
_____
_____
_____

Notes About:_____ Date: _/_/_

_____

_____

_____

_____

Notes About:_____ Date: _/_/_

_____

_____

_____

_____

Notes About:_____ Date: _/_/_

_____

_____

_____

_____

Notes About:_____ Date: _/_/_

_____

_____

_____

_____

Notes About:_____ Date: __/__/__

_____
_____
_____
_____

Notes About:_____ Date: __/__/__

_____
_____
_____
_____

Notes About:_____ Date: __/__/__

_____
_____
_____
_____

Notes About:_____ Date: __/__/__

_____
_____
_____
_____

Notes About:_____ Date: _/_/_

_____
_____
_____
_____

Notes About:_____ Date: _/_/_

_____
_____
_____
_____

Notes About:_____ Date: _/_/_

_____
_____
_____
_____

Notes About:_____ Date: _/_/_

_____
_____
_____
_____

Notes About:_____ Date: _/_/_

_____
_____
_____
_____

Notes About:_____ Date: _/_/_

_____
_____
_____
_____

Notes About:_____ Date: _/_/_

_____
_____
_____
_____

Notes About:_____ Date: _/_/_

_____
_____
_____
_____